LIVING WITH CHRONIC PAIN

Practical Solutions for a Pain-free Life with Proven Strategies, Treatments, and Therapies for Managing Long-Term Pain

Dr. Sarah J. Winters

Alpha Zuriel Publishing

Alpha Zuriel Publishing
Printed in the United States of America

Book Cover © 2024 Anchorage

Living with Chronic Pain -- 1st ed.

Disclaimer

The content provided in this book is for informational purposes only and is not intended to be a substitute for professional medical advice, diagnosis, or treatment. Every individual's situation is unique, and the general guidelines and recommendations may not apply to everyone. Consulting with a healthcare provider familiar with your specific situation is essential.

The information in this book is based on research and sources believed to be accurate and reliable at the time of publication. However, medical knowledge and guidelines change, and new research may emerge. Readers are encouraged to seek current information from reputable sources and consult with healthcare providers.

Any dietary or lifestyle changes, exercises, or other practices recommended in this book may carry potential risks and side effects. It is vital to consult with a healthcare provider who can assess individual risks and recommend appropriate actions.

The book is provided "as is" without any express or implied warranties. While efforts have been made to ensure accuracy and reliability, there is no guarantee that the information is error-free, complete, or suitable for any specific purpose.

Neither the authors nor publishers shall be liable for any loss, damage, injury, or adverse effects resulting from the application of the information contained in the book. Readers assume full responsibility for their use of the information.

The book may contain references to third-party websites, products, or services. These references are provided for convenience and do not constitute an endorsement or recommendation. The authors and publishers have no control over third-party content and are not responsible for its accuracy or reliability.

All content within the book is protected by copyright laws, and reproduction, distribution, or use without proper authorization is prohibited. Medical practices, dietary guidelines, and healthcare systems may vary across different cultures and regions, and readers should be aware of these variations when applying the information.

Some content in this book may be emotionally challenging or triggering for some readers. Engaging with the material with awareness of personal emotional responses and seeking support if needed is advisable.

The book is written in English and may not be accessible to all readers. Interpretations and translations should be handled with care, as nuances and specific meanings may be lost or altered.

This disclaimer emphasizes the importance of individual judgment, professional guidance, and personal responsibility when engaging with the content of the book. The information presented is intended to be informative and inspiring but must be used with caution and awareness of its limitations. By proceeding to read the book, readers acknowledge and accept the terms and conditions outlined in this disclaimer. It is the reader's responsibility to use the information within the book wisely and consult with appropriate medical and professional experts as needed.

Thank you for your understanding and happy reading!

CONTENTS

UNDERSTANDING CHRONIC PAIN 1

What is Chronic Pain and How it Affects Your Life 1

The Difference Between Acute and Chronic Pain 3

Why Managing Chronic Pain is About More Than Just Physical
Symptoms 4

IDENTIFYING THE CAUSES OF CHRONIC PAIN 7

Common Causes of Chronic Pain 7

Neuropathy, Nerve Damage, and Migraines 9

Post-Surgical Pain, Injuries, and Other Causes 10

How to Know What's Causing Your Pain 11

Diagnostic Tests and Medical Examinations 12

Working with Your Doctor to Find the Source of Your Pain 14

THE EMOTIONAL AND MENTAL IMPACT OF CHRONIC PAIN
.... 17

The Connection Between Chronic Pain, Anxiety, and Depression 17

Dealing with Emotional Exhaustion and Frustration 20

Coping with the Mental Challenges of Pain 21

Learning to Balance Your Emotions and Mental Health 23

Building Resilience Through Therapy and Support 24

MEDICAL TREATMENTS FOR PAIN RELIEF 25

Over-the-Counter Pain Relievers: NSAIDs, Acetaminophen 27

Prescription Medications: Opioids, Muscle Relaxants, and Anti-
Seizure Medications 29

Antidepressants for Pain: How They Help 31

Understanding Pain Medication Side Effects 32

Balancing Effectiveness and Safety in Long-Term Medication Use
.... 34

How to Work with Your Doctor to Manage Dosages 35

Injections and Nerve Blocks 37

Cortisone Injections, Nerve Blocks, and Other Interventions for Pain Relief..38

When Injections are the Best Option and What to Expect 40

ALTERNATIVE AND COMPLEMENTARY THERAPIES 43

How Exercise and Physical Therapy Help Manage Pain 44

Mind-Body Therapies...53

Meditation, Deep Breathing, and Relaxation Techniques.............55

LIFESTYLE CHANGES TO MANAGE CHRONIC PAIN 57

Diet and Nutrition for Pain Relief..57

Exercise for Pain Management 62

Improving Sleep with Chronic Pain..65

Managing Stress and Pain Together 67

COGNITIVE AND BEHAVIORAL APPROACHES TO PAIN 71

Cognitive Behavioral Therapy (CBT) 72

Acceptance and Commitment Therapy (ACT)..............................75

Biofeedback and Pain Management 77

LONG-TERM MANAGEMENT OF CHRONIC PAIN....................81

Building a Pain Management Plan...81

Tools for Tracking Pain, Symptoms, and Medication....................88

COPING WITH THE EMOTIONAL IMPACT OF PAIN 93

How to Cope When Pain Feels Overwhelming..............................95

Building a Positive Mindset in the Face of Chronic Pain..............97

The Role of Support Groups and Talking with Others Who Understand 99

Connecting with Chronic Pain Communities 100

How to Share Your Experience with Friends and Family............104

Working with a Therapist 105

CONCLUSION..108

Living Well with Chronic Pain..108

Appendices 113

UNDERSTANDING CHRONIC PAIN

What is Chronic Pain and How it Affects Your Life

Chronic pain is defined as any pain that persists for more than three to six months, often continuing long after the initial injury or illness has healed. It can result from a variety of conditions, including injury, arthritis, nerve damage, or illnesses like Lyme disease. Chronic pain is not just a physical sensation; it is a complex experience that impacts every aspect of an individual's life, including their emotional well-being, daily activities, and overall quality of life.

People suffering from chronic pain often find that it becomes a defining feature of their lives. The constant discomfort can make even the simplest activities—such as walking, sleeping, or sitting—feel exhausting and overwhelming. Chronic pain can lead to a cycle of inactivity, where physical limitations result in decreased movement, leading to muscle stiffness and further pain. This inactivity can spiral into feelings of frustration, isolation, and depression as the person struggles with a loss of independence.

Pain that lingers over a prolonged period can also strain personal relationships and professional life. Patients often experience difficulty explaining their condition to others, especially when there is no visible injury or clear medical explanation. This lack of understanding can lead to feelings of isolation, where the person feels that no one truly grasps the magnitude of their suffering. The psychological toll of chronic pain is immense, as it chips away at a person's confidence, hope, and sense of self.

The Difference Between Acute and Chronic Pain

Understanding the distinction between acute and chronic pain is crucial for developing an appropriate treatment approach. Acute pain is the body's natural response to injury or illness. It acts as a warning signal, alerting you to potential damage and encouraging you to rest or seek treatment. This type of pain is often short-lived, usually resolving once the underlying cause—such as a broken bone, cut, or infection—has healed.

In contrast, chronic pain persists long after the initial cause has resolved, and in many cases, no clear cause remains. It's no longer a warning signal but a persistent discomfort that becomes part of daily life. The body's pain signals remain active for months or even years, sometimes without any identifiable reason. While acute pain is generally associated with inflammation or injury, chronic pain can arise from a malfunction in the nervous system or as a result of long-term conditions like arthritis, fibromyalgia, or Lyme disease.

This difference is significant because while acute pain can usually be treated with rest, medication, and rehabilitation, chronic pain requires a more comprehensive and sustained approach. Simply addressing the physical symptoms is rarely enough. Effective chronic pain management often involves addressing emotional and psychological aspects, making it a far more complex condition to treat.

Why Managing Chronic Pain is About More Than Just Physical Symptoms

When dealing with chronic pain, focusing solely on the physical symptoms overlooks the broader, more profound effects the condition has on a person's overall well-being. Chronic pain is not just a physical sensation; it's an experience that deeply affects emotional and mental health. Over time, the constant strain of dealing with pain can lead to significant emotional distress, including anxiety, depression, and a sense of hopelessness.

The emotional toll of chronic pain can sometimes be as debilitating as the physical discomfort itself. Patients frequently report feelings of irritability, frustration, and sadness, stemming from their inability to perform daily tasks, maintain relationships, or enjoy hobbies. The constant struggle can lead to a negative feedback loop, where the pain exacerbates feelings of depression, and depression, in turn, heightens the perception of pain.

This relationship between the physical and emotional aspects of pain highlights the importance of a multidisciplinary approach to management. Pain is not simply a physical condition that can be treated with medication or physical therapy. Instead, it must be approached holistically, addressing both the body and the mind. Treatments like cognitive-behavioral therapy (CBT), mindfulness practices, and support groups can be essential components of a comprehensive pain management strategy. These methods help patients cope with the emotional and psychological burdens of chronic pain, enabling them to develop resilience and regain some control over their lives.

CHAPTER ONE

IDENTIFYING THE CAUSES OF CHRONIC PAIN

Common Causes of Chronic Pain

Arthritis, Fibromyalgia, and Back Pain

Arthritis is one of the leading causes of chronic pain, affecting millions of people worldwide. The most common forms include osteoarthritis and rheumatoid arthritis. Osteoarthritis results from the breakdown of cartilage, the tissue that cushions the ends of bones within joints, leading to pain, stiffness, and swelling. Rheumatoid arthritis, on the other hand, is an autoimmune disease where the immune system attacks the joints, causing inflammation, pain, and sometimes deformity.

Fibromyalgia is another condition known for widespread chronic pain. Unlike arthritis, fibromyalgia doesn't involve inflammation of the joints but instead is characterized by muscle pain, tenderness, and fatigue. The exact cause of fibromyalgia remains unclear, but researchers believe it involves a combination of genetic factors, infections, and physical or emotional trauma, all of which affect the way the brain processes pain signals.

Back pain, particularly lower back pain, is one of the most prevalent causes of chronic discomfort, often resulting from poor posture, injury, or degenerative changes in the spine. Conditions such as herniated discs, sciatica (pain radiating from the lower back down the legs due to nerve compression), and spinal stenosis (narrowing of the spinal canal) are frequent contributors to persistent back pain. Muscular problems, skeletal imbalances, or lifestyle factors like prolonged sitting can also play significant roles in chronic back pain.

Neuropathy, Nerve Damage, and Migraines

Neuropathy and nerve damage are significant causes of chronic pain, especially in individuals with diabetes, where diabetic neuropathy is a common complication. Neuropathy results from damage to the peripheral nerves, leading to sensations like tingling, numbness, burning, or sharp pain, usually in the hands and feet. Other causes of nerve damage can include traumatic injuries, infections, or exposure to toxins.

Migraines, another source of chronic pain, are severe headaches often accompanied by nausea, vomiting, and sensitivity to light or sound. Unlike typical tension headaches, migraines are thought to involve complex neurological changes, including alterations in blood flow to the brain. Chronic migraines—those that occur 15 or more days per month—can be debilitating, affecting daily life and work. While their exact cause isn't fully understood, genetic and environmental factors are believed to play key roles.

Post-Surgical Pain, Injuries, and Other Causes

Chronic pain can also develop after surgeries or injuries, a condition referred to as post-surgical pain syndrome or post-traumatic pain. For some individuals, pain persists long after the tissue damage from surgery or injury has healed. This could be due to nerve damage during surgery, inflammation, or the development of scar tissue. Conditions like complex regional pain syndrome (CRPS) can occur after an injury or surgery, leading to prolonged and severe pain, usually affecting a limb.

How to Know What's Causing Your Pain

Identifying the underlying cause of chronic pain can be a complex and lengthy process. Chronic pain is often multifaceted, meaning it may arise from more than one source or condition, complicating its diagnosis. In many cases, the cause is not immediately obvious and requires careful evaluation. Pinpointing the cause of chronic pain is essential to developing an effective treatment plan. Below, we explore the key diagnostic tools and approaches that help identify the source of chronic pain.

Diagnostic Tests and Medical Examinations

When you present with chronic pain, a thorough medical history and physical examination are the first steps in determining the cause. Your doctor will ask about the location, duration, and intensity of your pain, as well as any accompanying symptoms. They will also inquire about your lifestyle, previous injuries, surgeries, and any chronic conditions, such as arthritis or diabetes, that could be contributing factors.

Several diagnostic tests can be employed to gain further insights:

• Imaging tests such as X-rays, CT scans, and MRIs are used to visualize the bones, joints, muscles, and soft tissues. X-rays are typically useful in identifying structural issues like fractures or arthritis, while MRIs and CT scans offer more detailed images to detect soft tissue damage, herniated discs, or nerve impingement.

• Blood tests may be ordered if an autoimmune condition, such as rheumatoid arthritis or lupus, is suspected. These tests can reveal markers of inflammation, immune system activity, or the presence of specific antibodies linked to certain diseases.

• Nerve studies like electromyography (EMG) or nerve conduction studies are often used to detect neuropathy or nerve damage. These tests measure the electrical activity in muscles and the speed of nerve signals to assess how well your nerves are functioning.

- Bone scans or dual-energy X-ray absorptiometry (DEXA) scans may be used to identify conditions like osteoporosis or cancer that affect bone health, causing chronic pain.
- Diagnostic injections, such as nerve blocks or facet joint injections, can help pinpoint the source of pain by numbing specific areas. If your pain subsides after the injection, it provides valuable clues about the affected nerves or joints.

Working with Your Doctor to Find the Source of Your Pain

A key aspect of identifying the cause of chronic pain is effective communication with your healthcare provider. Chronic pain is often subjective and can vary greatly between individuals. Therefore, it is important to describe your pain as accurately and thoroughly as possible.

Some aspects to consider when discussing your pain with your doctor include:

- **Location:** Is your pain localized to a specific area, or does it radiate to other parts of your body?
- **Intensity:** How severe is your pain on a scale of 1 to 10? Does it fluctuate, or is it consistent throughout the day?
- **Nature:** Is your pain sharp, dull, throbbing, or burning? Different types of pain can point to different causes.
- **Duration:** How long have you experienced the pain? Did it begin suddenly, or has it gradually worsened over time?
- **Triggers:** Are there specific activities, movements, or positions that worsen or alleviate your pain?

A collaborative approach with your doctor will help in identifying patterns and narrowing down potential causes. Your doctor may also refer you to specialists, such as a rheumatologist for autoimmune diseases, a neurologist for nerve-related conditions, or an orthopedic surgeon for joint or spinal issues.

In cases where multiple causes are suspected, a multidisciplinary approach—involving pain specialists, physical therapists, and mental health professionals—may be necessary to comprehensively address the issue. Chronic pain often requires a team effort, as it can involve not only physical but also emotional and psychological components.

THE EMOTIONAL AND MENTAL IMPACT OF CHRONIC PAIN

The Connection Between Chronic Pain, Anxiety, and Depression

Pain is more than just a physical sensation. It involves complex signals that travel from the body to the brain, where they are processed and interpreted. When pain becomes chronic, it can change the way your brain perceives and responds to pain stimuli, making you more sensitive over time. This hypersensitivity can amplify not only physical pain but emotional responses as well.

Living with persistent pain often leads to negative emotional states such as irritability, sadness, and anger. It's common for people to feel overwhelmed or defeated, particularly when they've tried various treatments without finding relief. This emotional strain can build over time, affecting relationships with family, friends, and even healthcare providers. The frustration of not being able to engage fully in life's activities can lead to feelings of isolation and a loss of self-worth.

Moreover, the chronic nature of pain often disrupts sleep, leading to fatigue, which further impacts mood and cognitive function. Poor sleep can exacerbate feelings of sadness, confusion, and irritability, creating a cycle where pain and mood continually worsen each other. This interaction between pain and mood is why it's essential to recognize and address the emotional impact of chronic pain, rather than treating it solely as a physical condition.

Chronic pain and mental health disorders like anxiety and depression are often intertwined. Studies show that individuals living with chronic pain are significantly more likely to experience these conditions compared to the general population. In fact, up to 50% of people with chronic pain also suffer from depression, and anxiety is similarly prevalent.

Depression in the context of chronic pain often arises from a sense of hopelessness. When pain persists despite treatments, it can feel as though the body is betraying itself. The loss of control over one's physical well-being can manifest in feelings of despair, lack of motivation, and a decreased ability to enjoy life. Individuals may withdraw socially, lose interest in activities that once brought them joy, and experience overwhelming fatigue, all classic symptoms of depression.

Anxiety frequently accompanies chronic pain as well, particularly when the source of the pain is uncertain, or there is fear of exacerbating the condition. Worries about how pain will affect daily life, work, or relationships can build into a cycle of stress, which in turn can heighten the perception of pain. Anxiety also causes physical symptoms like muscle tension and rapid heart rate, which may intensify existing pain or even trigger new pain points.

The connection between pain, anxiety, and depression forms a vicious cycle: pain worsens mental health, and poor mental health exacerbates pain. This cycle is often referred to as the pain-depression-anxiety triad, and breaking it requires addressing both the physical and psychological aspects of chronic pain.

Dealing with Emotional Exhaustion and Frustration

One of the most challenging aspects of chronic pain is the ongoing emotional exhaustion it creates. Unlike acute pain, which has an identifiable cause and typically resolves with treatment, chronic pain can feel relentless. The continuous battle against pain, coupled with failed attempts to alleviate it, can drain emotional reserves, leaving individuals feeling mentally depleted.

This emotional exhaustion often leads to frustration. People with chronic pain may find themselves questioning why their body isn't healing or why treatments aren't working as expected. This frustration can be directed inward, resulting in self-blame, or outward, affecting relationships and interactions with others. Friends and family might not fully understand the depth of the pain or the mental toll it takes, leading to feelings of being misunderstood or dismissed.

Moreover, frustration can build when there is no clear diagnosis or when doctors are unable to find a specific cause for the pain. Not knowing what's wrong or how to fix it can lead to a sense of helplessness, further deepening emotional distress.

Coping with the Mental Challenges of Pain

Coping with the mental and emotional challenges of chronic pain requires a multi-faceted approach. It's important to acknowledge that pain is not just physical but also psychological, and that addressing both dimensions is crucial for effective management.

Some strategies for coping include:

• **Mindfulness and meditation:** These practices can help you develop an awareness of your body's pain signals and how they affect your thoughts and emotions. Mindfulness teaches individuals to observe their pain without judgment, which can reduce the emotional charge attached to it and make it easier to cope with.

• **Cognitive behavioral therapy (CBT):** CBT is a type of therapy that helps reframe negative thought patterns surrounding pain. It focuses on identifying and changing maladaptive thoughts and behaviors that may worsen pain, helping individuals adopt healthier ways of thinking and coping.

• **Physical activity:** While exercise may seem counterintuitive for those with chronic pain, gentle activities like yoga, swimming, or walking can help reduce pain and boost mood. Physical movement releases endorphins, the body's natural painkillers, and helps maintain mobility, reducing stiffness and discomfort.

• **Support groups:** Connecting with others who experience chronic pain can be immensely therapeutic.

Support groups offer a space to share experiences, vent frustrations, and learn coping strategies from those who truly understand the emotional and mental toll of pain.

Learning to Balance Your Emotions and Mental Health

Balancing emotions in the face of chronic pain can feel like a constant juggling act. It's essential to recognize that the emotional rollercoaster is a normal part of living with chronic pain, and learning to manage these feelings is key to long-term resilience.

One crucial strategy is practicing emotional regulation. This involves becoming aware of your emotional responses to pain and learning techniques to manage them effectively. For example, deep breathing exercises, progressive muscle relaxation, and guided imagery can help calm the nervous system and reduce the intensity of emotional reactions to pain.

Acceptance is another important aspect of emotional balance. It doesn't mean giving up on finding relief, but rather coming to terms with the reality of the pain and learning to live alongside it, without letting it dominate your mental and emotional well-being. This shift in perspective can help alleviate some of the frustration and hopelessness that often accompanies chronic pain.

Building Resilience Through Therapy and Support

Therapy plays a crucial role in helping individuals build resilience against the emotional and mental toll of chronic pain. Professional therapy, whether through a psychologist, psychiatrist, or licensed counselor, provides tools and techniques to manage both the physical and emotional aspects of pain.

Cognitive behavioral therapy (CBT), mentioned earlier, is especially effective in helping people with chronic pain. It helps individuals change the way they think about pain and develop coping strategies that reduce emotional distress. Other therapies, such as interpersonal therapy (IPT), can help improve relationships strained by the stress of chronic pain, while acceptance and commitment therapy (ACT) teaches individuals to accept their pain and commit to living a meaningful life despite it.

Finally, social support is vital for those with chronic pain. Whether through family, friends, or support groups, having a strong network of understanding individuals can provide both practical and emotional assistance. Sharing your experiences with others who know what it's like to live with chronic pain can be validating and reduce feelings of isolation.

CHAPTER THREE

MEDICAL TREATMENTS FOR PAIN RELIEF

Managing chronic pain often requires a multifaceted approach, including lifestyle changes, psychological therapies, and medical treatments. One of the most common and direct ways to address pain is through medication. While pain medications can offer significant relief, it's crucial to understand how each type works, the potential side effects, and the importance of balancing effectiveness with long-term safety.

Medications for Pain Management

Medications used to treat chronic pain can be divided into several categories, each targeting different pain mechanisms in the body. Some work by reducing inflammation, others alter the way the brain processes pain signals, and certain drugs even help calm the nervous system to reduce hypersensitivity. The right medication for each individual depends on the nature of the pain, its intensity, and any underlying conditions contributing to the pain.

It's important to remember that medications are not a one-size-fits-all solution. What works for one person may not work for another, and some medications may cause unwanted side effects. Therefore, it's essential to work closely with a healthcare provider to tailor a pain management plan that's both effective and safe.

Over-the-Counter Pain Relievers: NSAIDs, Acetaminophen

For mild to moderate pain, over-the-counter (OTC) medications are often the first line of treatment. Two of the most common categories of OTC pain relievers are nonsteroidal anti-inflammatory drugs (NSAIDs) and acetaminophen.

- **NSAIDs:** This class of drugs includes ibuprofen (Advil, Motrin), naproxen (Aleve), and aspirin. NSAIDs work by reducing inflammation, which is a common source of pain in conditions like arthritis, muscle strains, and tendonitis. By blocking the production of prostaglandins (chemicals that promote inflammation, pain, and fever), NSAIDs not only relieve pain but also reduce swelling and inflammation. These drugs are particularly useful for inflammatory conditions like osteoarthritis or injuries that cause swelling.

- **Acetaminophen (Tylenol):** Unlike NSAIDs, acetaminophen does not reduce inflammation. Instead, it works by altering the brain's perception of pain. Acetaminophen is often recommended for headaches, minor aches, and fevers. It is gentler on the stomach than NSAIDs, making it a safer option for individuals who may have gastrointestinal issues or ulcers.

While both NSAIDs and acetaminophen are effective for short-term use, long-term or excessive use can lead to complications. NSAIDs, for example, can increase the risk of gastrointestinal bleeding, kidney problems, and, in some cases, cardiovascular issues. Acetaminophen, if taken in high doses or combined with alcohol, can lead to liver damage. Therefore, these medications should be used according to the recommended dosages and only under the supervision of a healthcare provider for long-term pain management.

Prescription Medications: Opioids, Muscle Relaxants, and Anti-Seizure Medications

When OTC pain relievers are insufficient, doctors may prescribe stronger medications to manage more severe or persistent pain. Prescription pain medications come in several forms, each with distinct mechanisms of action and potential risks.

- **Opioids:** Opioids, such as oxycodone, hydrocodone, and morphine, are powerful pain relievers that work by binding to opioid receptors in the brain, altering the perception of pain. They are typically prescribed for acute pain (such as post-surgical pain) or chronic pain that does not respond to other treatments. While opioids can be effective for short-term use, they carry a high risk of addiction, dependence, and overdose. Prolonged use can also lead to tolerance, where the body requires higher doses to achieve the same level of pain relief. Because of these risks, opioids are generally reserved for severe pain that cannot be managed with other treatments, and they are prescribed with caution.

- **Muscle relaxants:** These medications, such as cyclobenzaprine (Flexeril) or baclofen, are often prescribed for muscle-related pain, such as that caused by muscle spasms or tension. Muscle relaxants work by reducing muscle tone, relieving stiffness, and easing discomfort associated with muscle injuries or conditions like fibromyalgia. However, they can cause drowsiness, dizziness, and dry mouth, so they are often recommended for short-term use or under strict medical supervision.

- **Anti-seizure medications:** Drugs originally developed to treat epilepsy, such as gabapentin (Neurontin) and pregabalin (Lyrica), have also been found effective for certain types of chronic pain, especially nerve pain or neuropathy. These medications work by calming overactive nerves, reducing the abnormal pain signals they send to the brain. This makes them particularly useful for conditions like diabetic neuropathy, postherpetic neuralgia (shingles pain), or fibromyalgia. Side effects may include dizziness, fatigue, and weight gain, so regular monitoring is necessary.

Antidepressants for Pain: How They Help

Interestingly, some types of antidepressants are also used to manage chronic pain. Medications such as tricyclic antidepressants (TCAs), including amitriptyline, and serotonin-norepinephrine reuptake inhibitors (SNRIs), like duloxetine (Cymbalta) and venlafaxine, have been shown to alleviate certain types of pain, particularly neuropathic pain and fibromyalgia.

These medications work by altering the levels of neurotransmitters—specifically serotonin and norepinephrine—in the brain, which can influence how pain signals are processed. By boosting these chemicals, antidepressants can reduce the perception of pain and improve mood, which is often affected by chronic pain. The dual benefit of addressing both pain and the emotional toll it takes makes these drugs a valuable part of chronic pain treatment plans.

It's important to note that antidepressants used for pain are not prescribed because the pain is "all in your head." These medications have direct effects on the nervous system's ability to process pain signals, making them effective even in cases where no underlying depression exists.

Understanding Pain Medication Side Effects

All pain medications, whether over-the-counter or prescription, come with potential side effects. Understanding and monitoring these side effects is essential to ensuring safe and effective pain management.

- **NSAIDs:** Common side effects include gastrointestinal issues such as stomach pain, ulcers, and bleeding. Long-term use can lead to kidney damage and increase the risk of heart attack or stroke.

- **Acetaminophen:** Overuse of acetaminophen can cause liver damage, especially when taken in high doses or combined with alcohol. It's crucial to stay within the recommended daily limit, typically no more than 4,000 milligrams for adults.

- **Opioids:** The most concerning side effects of opioids are respiratory depression, constipation, drowsiness, and the risk of addiction or dependence. Long-term use can also lead to tolerance, where the body requires higher doses for the same pain relief, further increasing the risk of overdose.

- **Muscle relaxants:** These can cause drowsiness, dizziness, dry mouth, and confusion, particularly in older adults. They are generally not recommended for long-term use due to these risks.

- **Anti-seizure medications:** Common side effects include dizziness, fatigue, and weight gain. Some individuals may experience mood changes, including depression or suicidal thoughts, so close monitoring by a healthcare provider is necessary.

- **Antidepressants:** In addition to their benefits for pain, antidepressants can cause side effects like dry mouth, drowsiness, weight gain, and sexual dysfunction. In some cases, they may also worsen anxiety or depression before improvements are seen, so it's important to report any changes in mood to your doctor.

Balancing Effectiveness and Safety in Long-Term Medication Use

For individuals with chronic pain, long-term medication use may be necessary to maintain quality of life. However, it's essential to balance the effectiveness of the medication with the potential risks, particularly when it comes to side effects or dependency. This is why a comprehensive, individualized pain management plan is critical.

Healthcare providers will often start with the least invasive treatments, such as OTC pain relievers or physical therapy, and gradually introduce stronger medications only when necessary. Regular follow-ups are crucial for monitoring the effectiveness of medications, adjusting dosages, or switching to different treatments if side effects become intolerable or if the pain worsens.

In some cases, multimodal therapy—using a combination of medications and other treatments such as physical therapy, acupuncture, or cognitive behavioral therapy—can reduce the need for higher doses of medications, minimizing the risk of side effects while still providing effective pain relief.

Patients should always communicate openly with their healthcare providers about how they are responding to medications, any side effects they experience, and their overall goals for pain management. This collaborative approach ensures that pain management is not only effective but also sustainable in the long term.

How to Work with Your Doctor to Manage Dosages

When it comes to managing chronic pain, one of the most critical aspects is finding the correct dosage of medication. Striking the right balance between effectiveness and safety can be a challenge, particularly with long-term medication use. Working closely with your doctor is essential to ensuring that your dosages provide sufficient pain relief without causing unnecessary side effects or leading to dependence.

The dosage of any medication, whether it's an over-the-counter pain reliever, a prescription opioid, or an antidepressant, needs to be carefully adjusted based on your response and the severity of your pain. Here are some key considerations when working with your doctor to manage dosages:

Start Low, Go Slow: In many cases, doctors will begin with the lowest possible dose of a medication and increase it gradually if needed. This allows them to monitor how well the medication is working and minimize the risk of side effects. It's important to be patient with this process, as it may take time to find the optimal dose.

Communicate Regularly: Open communication with your doctor is vital. Keep them informed about how well the medication is controlling your pain, any side effects you're experiencing, and how the medication affects your daily life. For example, if you notice that your pain flares up at certain times of the day or after specific activities, your doctor may adjust your dosage schedule to provide more consistent relief.

Monitor for Tolerance: Over time, some medications, particularly opioids, can lead to tolerance, where the same dose becomes less effective and higher doses are required for the same level of pain relief. If you feel that your medication is becoming less effective, it's important to discuss this with your doctor rather than increasing the dose on your own. Your doctor may adjust the medication, introduce a new treatment, or explore alternative pain management options.

Consider Medication Rotation: In some cases, rotating between different classes of medications can help maintain effectiveness without increasing the dosage of any single drug. For example, alternating between an NSAID and acetaminophen can provide pain relief without the need for higher doses of either medication.

Tapering Off Medications: If you've been taking a medication for a long time and are considering stopping, it's essential to do so under your doctor's guidance. Certain medications, particularly opioids and antidepressants, should be tapered off gradually to avoid withdrawal symptoms or the sudden return of pain. Your doctor can help develop a tapering schedule that minimizes discomfort.

Non-Medication Strategies: While medication is a key component of pain management, it's also important to explore non-medication strategies such as physical therapy, relaxation techniques, or cognitive behavioral therapy. By combining medications with other treatments, you may be able to lower the dosage while still achieving effective pain relief.

Injections and Nerve Blocks

For some individuals, oral medications may not be sufficient to manage chronic pain, or the side effects of these medications may outweigh the benefits. In such cases, doctors may recommend injections or nerve blocks as an alternative or supplementary treatment. These minimally invasive procedures target specific areas of pain and can provide longer-lasting relief than oral medications.

Cortisone Injections, Nerve Blocks, and Other Interventions for Pain Relief

Cortisone injections are one of the most common types of injections used to relieve pain, particularly for conditions involving inflammation, such as arthritis, bursitis, and tendonitis. Cortisone is a powerful anti-inflammatory steroid that, when injected directly into the site of pain, can reduce inflammation and provide pain relief for weeks or even months.

Cortisone injections are often used for joint pain, particularly in the knees, hips, and shoulders. They can also be helpful for conditions like carpal tunnel syndrome, where inflammation of the tendons causes nerve compression. While cortisone injections can be highly effective, they should not be overused, as repeated injections can weaken tendons and cartilage over time.

Nerve blocks are another type of injection used to target chronic pain. These injections involve the use of an anesthetic or anti-inflammatory medication to block pain signals from a specific nerve or group of nerves. Nerve blocks are particularly useful for treating neuropathic pain, such as sciatica or pain from a herniated disc. They can also be used for conditions like complex regional pain syndrome (CRPS) or migraines that don't respond well to other treatments.

Other types of injections include trigger point injections, which target areas of muscle pain known as trigger points, and hyaluronic acid injections, often used to relieve knee pain in individuals with osteoarthritis by providing lubrication to the joint.

When Injections are the Best Option and What to Expect

Injections are typically considered when oral medications or other conservative treatments fail to provide adequate relief. They are especially beneficial for individuals with localized pain, where targeting a specific area with medication can provide significant relief with fewer systemic side effects.

Your doctor may recommend injections if you:

- Have pain that is localized to a specific joint, nerve, or muscle

- Have tried other treatments, such as oral medications or physical therapy, without success

- Are looking for longer-lasting pain relief than what oral medications provide

- Have pain that is caused by inflammation, nerve damage, or specific musculoskeletal issues

What to Expect:

Before the injection, your doctor will explain the procedure, including any potential risks or side effects. Depending on the type of injection, you may receive a local anesthetic to numb the area.

During the injection, you might feel pressure or discomfort as the needle is inserted, but the procedure is generally quick. For some injections, such as those guided by imaging (e.g., ultrasound or X-ray), the doctor will use real-time imaging to ensure the medication is delivered to the precise location.

After the injection, you may experience soreness at the injection site for a few days, but this usually subsides quickly. Pain relief can begin within a few days and may last for weeks or months, depending on the type of injection and the underlying condition.

It's important to follow your doctor's post-procedure instructions, which may include rest, ice application, or avoiding certain activities. While injections can provide significant relief, they are usually part of a broader pain management plan that may also include physical therapy or lifestyle changes to maintain mobility and reduce the risk of future pain.

CHAPTER FOUR

ALTERNATIVE AND COMPLEMENTARY THERAPIES

As the understanding of chronic pain deepens, many individuals are turning to alternative and complementary therapies to supplement traditional medical treatments. These therapies often focus on improving overall well-being, reducing stress, and addressing the underlying causes of pain from a holistic perspective. They can be particularly beneficial when combined with conventional treatments, offering relief without the side effects associated with medications.

Physical Therapy and Movement

Physical therapy (PT) is one of the most commonly recommended complementary therapies for managing chronic pain. It involves a range of techniques, including therapeutic exercises, manual therapies, and modalities like heat or cold therapy, all designed to improve mobility, strength, and function. The primary goal of physical therapy is to restore movement and function in the affected areas, alleviate pain, and prevent future injury.

How Exercise and Physical Therapy Help Manage Pain

Chronic pain often leads to decreased physical activity, which can result in weakened muscles, reduced flexibility, and worsened pain over time. Physical therapy helps break this cycle by gradually reintroducing safe, targeted movements that improve muscle strength and joint flexibility, promoting better overall function.

Exercise increases blood flow to muscles and joints, enhancing the healing process and reducing stiffness. Physical therapy also focuses on correcting posture, body mechanics, and movement patterns, which can alleviate pain caused by poor alignment or repetitive stress. For example, individuals with chronic back pain may benefit from exercises that strengthen the core muscles, providing better support for the spine and reducing strain.

Movement therapy can also help calm the nervous system, reducing the intensity of pain signals sent to the brain. Techniques such as manual therapy—where a physical therapist uses their hands to mobilize muscles and joints— can help alleviate muscle tension, improve range of motion, and decrease pain.

Safe and Gentle Exercises for People with Chronic Pain

When it comes to chronic pain, it's important to start with gentle, low-impact exercises that don't strain the body. Physical therapists often recommend:

Stretching exercises: Gentle stretching can improve flexibility and reduce stiffness in muscles and joints. Stretching is particularly beneficial for individuals with arthritis or fibromyalgia, as it helps maintain joint mobility and reduces the risk of injury.

Water-based exercises: Exercising in water reduces the impact on joints and provides natural resistance, making it an excellent option for people with conditions like osteoarthritis or fibromyalgia. Water aerobics or swimming can improve strength, endurance, and flexibility without placing stress on painful joints.

Low-impact aerobic exercises: Activities such as walking, cycling, or using an elliptical machine can increase cardiovascular health, improve circulation, and release endorphins—natural pain-relieving chemicals in the brain.

Strength training: Light resistance exercises using bands, light weights, or body weight can help build muscle without overloading the joints. Strengthening muscles around painful areas, such as the back or knees, can provide better support and reduce pain.

A physical therapist will design an individualized exercise program tailored to your specific needs and pain levels. It's important to start slowly, listen to your body, and avoid pushing through pain. Consistency and gradual progress are key to long-term improvement.

Acupuncture and Acupressure

Acupuncture and acupressure are traditional Chinese therapies that have been used for thousands of years to treat pain. These therapies are based on the belief that the body has energy channels, or meridians, that can become blocked or imbalanced, leading to pain and illness. By stimulating specific points on the body, acupuncture and acupressure are thought to restore balance and promote healing.

How These Traditional Therapies Provide Pain Relief

Acupuncture involves the insertion of thin, sterile needles into specific points on the body, known as acupoints. These needles stimulate the nervous system, triggering the release of endorphins, serotonin, and other natural pain-relieving chemicals. Acupuncture is also believed to improve circulation and reduce inflammation, making it an effective treatment for a variety of chronic pain conditions, including back pain, osteoarthritis, migraines, and fibromyalgia. Acupressure, which involves applying pressure to the same acupoints used in acupuncture, provides similar benefits without the use of needles. By pressing on specific points, acupressure helps to release muscle tension, improve blood flow, and reduce pain. It is often used for conditions like tension headaches, neck pain, and muscle soreness. Studies have shown that acupuncture and acupressure can be effective in reducing pain, improving function, and enhancing the overall quality of life for people with chronic pain. While these therapies may not completely eliminate pain, they can be a valuable component of a comprehensive pain management plan.

What to Expect from an Acupuncture Session

During an acupuncture session, a licensed practitioner will evaluate your condition, discuss your symptoms, and identify the specific points that will be targeted. Once the points are selected, the practitioner will gently insert very fine needles into your skin at these locations.

Most people experience little to no discomfort during the procedure, and the needles are usually left in place for 15-30 minutes. You may feel a mild tingling or a sensation of warmth around the needle sites, which is considered a positive sign that the treatment is stimulating the body's energy pathways.

After the session, some people report immediate pain relief, while others may notice improvement after a few treatments. Acupuncture is generally considered safe when performed by a trained professional, but it's important to choose a licensed practitioner to ensure proper technique and hygiene.

Massage Therapy and Chiropractic Care

Massage therapy and chiropractic care are two hands-on treatments that can be highly effective for managing muscle and joint pain. Both therapies focus on improving the function of the musculoskeletal system, but they do so through different techniques.

The Benefits of Hands-On Therapies for Muscle and Joint Pain

Massage therapy involves the manipulation of soft tissues, such as muscles, tendons, and ligaments, to improve circulation, relieve tension, and promote relaxation. For individuals with chronic pain, massage can help reduce muscle stiffness, improve range of motion, and alleviate stress, which is often a contributor to pain.

Regular massage sessions can also promote the release of endorphins, helping to reduce the perception of pain. It's especially useful for conditions like fibromyalgia, where muscle tenderness and tightness are common, as well as chronic back or neck pain caused by tension or poor posture. Chiropractic care focuses on the alignment of the spine and musculoskeletal system. Chiropractors use manual adjustments, or spinal manipulations, to correct misalignments in the spine (known as subluxations) that may be contributing to pain. By realigning the spine, chiropractic care aims to relieve pressure on nerves, reduce inflammation, and improve mobility.

When Chiropractic Adjustments Can Help with Chronic Pain

Chiropractic adjustments are most commonly used to treat conditions like back pain, neck pain, and headaches. They can also be beneficial for individuals with joint pain, such as in the knees or hips, by improving overall posture and body mechanics.

Chiropractic care is particularly effective for mechanical pain—pain caused by movement or positioning issues—where restoring proper alignment can reduce strain on muscles and joints. While chiropractic care is generally safe, it's important to seek treatment from a licensed chiropractor, especially if you have any underlying health conditions.

Mind-Body Therapies

Yoga, Tai Chi, and Other Mindful Movement Practices

Yoga and tai chi are two of the most well-known forms of mindful movement. Both practices focus on gentle, flowing movements combined with deep, controlled breathing and meditation. These mind-body exercises are particularly effective for individuals with chronic pain because they are low-impact and can be modified to suit a range of abilities and pain levels.

Yoga incorporates stretching, strength-building poses, and breath control (known as pranayama) to increase flexibility, balance, and mental focus. For people with chronic pain, yoga has been shown to reduce pain intensity, improve physical function, and enhance overall quality of life. Additionally, the mindfulness aspect of yoga can help individuals develop a greater awareness of their bodies and pain triggers, making it easier to manage discomfort.

Tai chi, on the other hand, is a form of martial art that involves slow, deliberate movements designed to promote relaxation and balance. Tai chi focuses on the connection between mind and body and can be particularly beneficial for individuals with conditions like fibromyalgia or arthritis. Studies have shown that regular tai chi practice can reduce pain, improve balance, and enhance mental well-being in people with chronic pain.

Both yoga and tai chi provide a gentle way to engage the body without exacerbating pain, making them ideal for those looking to incorporate movement into their pain management plan while also addressing the mental and emotional aspects of living with chronic pain.

Meditation, Deep Breathing, and Relaxation Techniques

Meditation and deep breathing exercises are foundational mind-body techniques that focus on calming the mind and reducing the body's stress response. Chronic pain often leads to heightened stress and anxiety, which can increase the perception of pain. By incorporating relaxation techniques into daily life, individuals can reduce this stress and cultivate a greater sense of calm, which in turn can alleviate pain. Meditation, particularly mindfulness meditation, encourages individuals to focus on the present moment and observe their thoughts, feelings, and sensations without judgment. This practice helps patients with chronic pain accept their condition and reduce emotional distress. Meditation can help break the cycle of pain and anxiety by training the mind to respond to pain in a less reactive and more controlled manner.

Deep breathing exercises work by activating the parasympathetic nervous system, which is responsible for the body's rest-and-digest response. When practiced regularly, deep breathing can lower heart rate, reduce muscle tension, and increase oxygen flow throughout the body, leading to a calming effect. Techniques like diaphragmatic breathing, where the breath is drawn deeply into the belly rather than shallowly into the chest, can be particularly helpful for managing pain flare-ups.

Other relaxation techniques, such as progressive muscle relaxation and guided imagery, involve consciously releasing tension from muscles or visualizing peaceful, calming scenarios. These practices not only help reduce pain but also improve overall mental health, providing an effective way to manage both the physical and emotional challenges of chronic pain.

CHAPTER FIVE

LIFESTYLE CHANGES TO MANAGE CHRONIC PAIN

Managing chronic pain often requires more than just medical treatments or medications. Making adjustments to your daily lifestyle can have a significant impact on reducing pain and improving your overall quality of life. Incorporating healthy habits such as a nutritious diet, regular physical activity, better sleep hygiene, and stress management can all contribute to better pain control and enhance physical and emotional well-being.

Diet and Nutrition for Pain Relief

The connection between diet and chronic pain is becoming increasingly clear. The food you eat can either help reduce inflammation or worsen it, making dietary choices a key component of managing chronic pain. By focusing on an anti-inflammatory diet, you can reduce the levels of chronic inflammation in your body, which is a common contributor to many painful conditions such as arthritis, fibromyalgia, and autoimmune disorders.

Anti-Inflammatory Foods to Include in Your Diet

Certain foods have natural anti-inflammatory properties that can help soothe pain and promote healing. A well-rounded diet that includes these foods can not only improve your pain levels but also support overall health and well-being. Key anti-inflammatory foods to incorporate into your diet include:

Fatty fish: Fish like salmon, mackerel, sardines, and tuna are rich in omega-3 fatty acids, which have been shown to reduce inflammation. Omega-3s can help alleviate joint pain, particularly in individuals with rheumatoid arthritis.

Leafy greens: Vegetables such as spinach, kale, and broccoli are packed with vitamins, minerals, and antioxidants that combat inflammation. They are also rich in fiber, which promotes gut health, another factor in reducing inflammation.

Berries: Blueberries, strawberries, and other berries are loaded with antioxidants that help fight free radicals, which are molecules that cause inflammation and damage to tissues. The anthocyanins in berries are particularly effective in reducing inflammatory markers.

Nuts and seeds: Almonds, walnuts, flaxseeds, and chia seeds are excellent sources of anti-inflammatory omega-3 fatty acids, as well as protein and fiber. They can help reduce inflammation and support heart and brain health.

Olive oil: Rich in oleocanthal, a compound with anti-inflammatory effects, extra virgin olive oil has been compared to NSAIDs for its ability to reduce pain and inflammation. Use it as a healthy fat option in cooking or salad dressings.

Turmeric: This bright yellow spice contains curcumin, a powerful anti-inflammatory and antioxidant compound. Turmeric has been studied extensively for its role in reducing pain, especially in individuals with arthritis.

Ginger: Known for its anti-inflammatory and analgesic properties, ginger can help relieve pain caused by muscle soreness, osteoarthritis, and inflammatory conditions.

By incorporating these foods into your diet, you can take a proactive step toward managing pain through nutrition.

Foods That Can Worsen Inflammation and Pain

Just as certain foods can reduce inflammation, others can exacerbate it, worsening pain and making it harder to manage chronic conditions. Foods that promote inflammation should be minimized or avoided, especially if you're struggling with chronic pain. These include:

Processed foods: Foods high in refined sugars, unhealthy fats, and preservatives—such as fast food, chips, and sugary snacks—can increase inflammation. These foods trigger spikes in blood sugar levels, leading to inflammatory responses in the body.

Sugary beverages: Sodas, energy drinks, and sweetened fruit juices are loaded with refined sugars that contribute to inflammation and can worsen conditions like joint pain or fibromyalgia.

Red and processed meats: High consumption of red meats (such as beef, pork, and lamb) and processed meats (like sausages, bacon, and hot dogs) has been linked to increased inflammation due to the presence of saturated fats and advanced glycation end products (AGEs), which can cause inflammatory responses.

Alcohol: Excessive alcohol consumption can increase inflammation in the body and contribute to joint pain, especially in individuals with arthritis. Alcohol can also interfere with sleep, which is crucial for pain management.

Trans fats: Found in many processed and fried foods, trans fats are known to increase inflammation and contribute to the development of chronic diseases. Reading labels and avoiding foods with "partially hydrogenated oils" can help reduce your intake of trans fats.

Eliminating or reducing these inflammatory foods can make a noticeable difference in your pain levels and overall health.

Exercise for Pain Management

The Benefits of Regular Physical Activity in Reducing Pain

Exercise has a wide range of benefits for those with chronic pain:

- **Improved mobility:** Regular exercise helps maintain joint flexibility and range of motion, reducing stiffness and improving mobility.

- **Stronger muscles:** Strengthening the muscles that support joints and the spine can help alleviate pain by providing more stability and reducing strain on affected areas.

- **Endorphin release:** Physical activity triggers the release of endorphins, hormones that act as natural painkillers and mood enhancers. This can help reduce pain and improve emotional well-being.

- **Reduced inflammation:** Exercise can reduce inflammation by improving circulation and promoting the body's natural healing processes.

- **Better sleep:** Regular physical activity can improve sleep quality, which is crucial for managing pain and promoting overall health.

While some pain sufferers may worry that exercise will worsen their symptoms, the key is to start slowly and choose activities that are safe and suitable for your condition.

Low-Impact Workouts: Swimming, Walking, and Stretching

Low-impact workouts are ideal for individuals with chronic pain, as they provide the benefits of physical activity without placing undue stress on joints and muscles. Some of the best low-impact exercises include:

• **Swimming:** Water-based exercises like swimming and water aerobics are particularly gentle on the joints because the water's buoyancy reduces the impact on the body. Swimming also provides a full-body workout that strengthens muscles and improves cardiovascular health.

• **Walking:** Walking is one of the simplest and most accessible forms of exercise. It improves circulation, strengthens muscles, and promotes joint flexibility. Start with short walks and gradually increase the duration and intensity as your stamina improves.

• **Stretching:** Stretching exercises help maintain flexibility and prevent stiffness, which is especially important for individuals with conditions like arthritis or fibromyalgia. Regular stretching can also improve posture and reduce muscle tension, both of which can help alleviate pain.

By incorporating these low-impact exercises into your routine, you can enjoy the benefits of physical activity without exacerbating your chronic pain.

Improving Sleep with Chronic Pain

Why Pain Can Affect Your Sleep and How to Sleep Better

Chronic pain often disrupts sleep for several reasons. Pain can make it difficult to find a comfortable sleeping position, leading to tossing and turning throughout the night. In some cases, pain may flare up during the night, waking you from sleep or preventing you from falling back asleep. Additionally, the stress and anxiety that often accompany chronic pain can make it harder to relax and drift off to sleep.

To improve sleep with chronic pain, consider the following strategies:

- **Create a comfortable sleep environment:** Invest in a supportive mattress and pillows that help reduce pressure on painful areas. Experiment with different sleep positions to find the one that is most comfortable for you.

- **Establish a sleep routine:** Go to bed and wake up at the same time every day, even on weekends. A consistent sleep schedule can help regulate your body's internal clock and improve sleep quality.

- **Practice relaxation techniques:** Deep breathing exercises, progressive muscle relaxation, or meditation before bed can help calm the mind and body, making it easier to fall asleep.

• **Limit caffeine and alcohol:** Both caffeine and alcohol can interfere with sleep quality, so try to avoid consuming them in the hours leading up to bedtime.

By implementing these practical strategies, you can improve your sleep and better manage your chronic pain.

Practical Tips for Getting Quality Rest While Managing Pain

1. **Sleep hygiene:** Establishing good sleep hygiene is key to getting restful sleep. Keep your bedroom dark, quiet, and cool, and avoid stimulating activities like watching TV or using electronic devices before bed.

2. **Pain management before bed:** Take steps to manage your pain before going to bed, such as applying heat or ice packs, using a topical pain reliever, or taking any prescribed medications.

3. **Gentle stretches before bed:** Performing gentle stretching exercises before bed can help release tension in muscles and joints, making it easier to relax and fall asleep.

4. **Consider a body pillow:** A body pillow can help provide support and alleviate pressure on painful areas, making it easier to find a comfortable sleeping position.

By making sleep a priority and taking steps to manage your pain at night, you can improve the quality of your rest and, as a result, better manage your chronic pain during the day.

Managing Stress and Pain Together

Stress and chronic pain often go hand-in-hand. Pain can increase stress levels, and stress can heighten pain sensitivity by triggering the body's fight-or-flight response. This stress response leads to the release of cortisol and other stress hormones that increase inflammation and exacerbate pain.

How Stress Can Increase Pain Sensitivity

When the body is under stress, the nervous system becomes hyperactive, which can amplify pain signals and make pain feel more intense. Prolonged stress can also cause muscle tension, particularly in the neck, shoulders, and back, leading to increased pain in these areas. Moreover, stress-related sleep disturbances can further exacerbate pain, making it harder to manage.

Learning to manage stress is key to breaking the cycle of pain and emotional distress.

Simple Stress-Reduction Techniques to Support Pain Relief

Managing stress can have a positive impact on both physical and emotional well-being. Some effective stress-reduction techniques include:

Mindfulness meditation: Mindfulness encourages being present in the moment without judgment. For chronic pain sufferers, mindfulness can be an effective way to focus on the here and now, rather than being consumed by worries about pain or future discomfort. Regular mindfulness practice can help shift the focus away from pain and reduce stress levels.

Physical activity: Exercise is one of the best ways to manage stress and pain simultaneously. Physical activity releases endorphins, natural chemicals that boost mood and reduce pain perception. Even gentle activities like walking, yoga, or tai chi can have significant benefits for both your physical and emotional well-being.

Hobbies and relaxation: Engaging in hobbies or activities that bring you joy can help distract from pain and reduce stress. Whether it's reading, gardening, painting, or knitting, dedicating time to enjoyable activities can promote relaxation and help you regain a sense of control over your life.

Time management and setting boundaries: Stress often stems from feeling overwhelmed or overcommitted. Learn to manage your time effectively by setting realistic goals and boundaries. Prioritize activities that support your health and well-being, and don't hesitate to say no to demands that may increase stress or pain.

By incorporating these stress-reduction techniques into your daily routine, you can better manage both the physical and emotional aspects of chronic pain. Reducing stress not only helps improve mood and mental health but can also decrease pain sensitivity, making it an important part of a comprehensive pain management strategy.

CHAPTER SIX

COGNITIVE AND BEHAVIORAL APPROACHES TO PAIN

Chronic pain doesn't just affect the body—it also impacts mental and emotional well-being. The mind and body are deeply interconnected, and this relationship plays a critical role in how we perceive and cope with pain. Cognitive and behavioral approaches, such as Cognitive Behavioral Therapy (CBT), Acceptance and Commitment Therapy (ACT), and biofeedback, offer powerful tools to help manage both the physical and emotional aspects of chronic pain. These therapies aim to shift negative thought patterns, improve emotional responses, and increase a sense of control over pain.

Cognitive Behavioral Therapy (CBT)

This is one of the most widely used psychological approaches for managing chronic pain. This form of therapy is based on the idea that thoughts, feelings, and behaviors are interconnected, and that by changing negative thought patterns, you can influence how you experience and respond to pain. CBT is highly effective for reducing the emotional distress associated with chronic pain and can help individuals develop healthier coping mechanisms.

How CBT Helps You Manage Negative Thoughts About Pain

Chronic pain often leads to negative, automatic thoughts such as, "I'll never get better," or "This pain is ruining my life." These thoughts can intensify feelings of hopelessness, anxiety, and depression, which in turn can amplify the perception of pain. CBT helps individuals recognize these negative thoughts and reframe them into more realistic, positive ones.

For example, instead of thinking, "I can't do anything because of my pain," CBT encourages a shift in perspective to, "There are still activities I can enjoy, even if I have to make adjustments." By challenging and changing negative thought patterns, CBT helps reduce the emotional suffering that accompanies chronic pain, leading to improved mood and a greater sense of control.

CBT also addresses catastrophizing—the tendency to predict the worst possible outcome, which is common in individuals with chronic pain. Learning to break this cycle of negative thinking can significantly reduce the intensity of pain and the emotional toll it takes.

Building Healthier Emotional Responses to Pain

Pain is not only a physical sensation but also an emotional experience. CBT teaches individuals how to build healthier emotional responses to pain by focusing on adaptive coping strategies. For example, when pain flares up, instead of reacting with frustration or anger, CBT encourages a mindful approach that involves acceptance, relaxation, and problem-solving.

Therapists may also introduce techniques like graded exposure, which helps people gradually face activities they have been avoiding due to pain. This reduces fear and anxiety related to pain and empowers individuals to engage more fully in life despite their condition.

Acceptance and Commitment Therapy (ACT)

While CBT focuses on changing negative thoughts, Acceptance and Commitment Therapy (ACT) takes a different approach. ACT encourages individuals to accept their pain, rather than fighting against it, while simultaneously committing to living a meaningful life despite the pain. Acceptance doesn't mean giving up on finding relief; rather, it involves acknowledging that pain may be a part of life and learning to cope with it in a way that allows for personal growth and fulfillment.

Learning to Accept Your Pain While Building a Full Life

At the core of ACT is the idea that struggling against pain can sometimes cause more suffering than the pain itself. When individuals are constantly trying to avoid or suppress their pain, they may end up feeling trapped, frustrated, and disconnected from the activities and people that bring them joy. ACT teaches people how to accept the presence of pain without letting it dominate their lives.

ACT encourages individuals to identify their core values—the things that matter most to them, such as family, career, or hobbies—and to take steps toward living in alignment with those values, even when pain is present. This shift in focus, from pain to values, can be incredibly empowering and helps reduce the emotional burden of chronic pain.

How to Focus on What Matters Most Despite Pain

ACT promotes the use of mindfulness techniques to stay grounded in the present moment. By practicing mindfulness, individuals can observe their pain without judgment and without becoming overwhelmed by it. Mindfulness helps people focus on the things that truly matter in their lives, rather than fixating on the pain.

For example, someone who values spending time with family might learn to engage in family activities, even on days when pain is more intense. Instead of focusing on the discomfort, they focus on the joy of being with loved ones, thus improving their quality of life despite the pain.

ACT encourages people to pursue meaningful activities and relationships, even in the presence of pain. This approach can lead to greater emotional resilience and a sense of accomplishment, as individuals learn that pain does not have to define or limit their lives.

Biofeedback and Pain Management

Biofeedback is a technique that helps individuals gain control over certain bodily functions that are typically involuntary, such as heart rate, muscle tension, or skin temperature. In the context of chronic pain, biofeedback can be used to help individuals become more aware of how their bodies react to stress, tension, and pain, and to teach them how to regulate these responses.

Using Biofeedback to Understand and Control Your Body's Response to Pain

Biofeedback works by using sensors attached to the skin to monitor physiological functions such as muscle tension, heart rate, and skin temperature. The information is then displayed on a monitor, allowing individuals to see how their bodies are responding in real-time. Through this feedback, people can learn to recognize how stress or anxiety might be affecting their pain levels.

For example, muscle tension is often a significant contributor to pain, particularly in conditions like back pain, migraines, or fibromyalgia. By observing how tension builds in certain muscles, individuals can learn to consciously relax those muscles, reducing both tension and pain. Similarly, learning to control heart rate or breathing patterns can help reduce the body's stress response, which can also alleviate pain.

Biofeedback provides a tangible way for individuals to see the connection between their mental state and their physical pain. This can be empowering, as it gives individuals greater control over their pain and the ability to actively influence their body's responses.

How to Use Biofeedback at Home to Relieve Tension

While biofeedback is often conducted in a clinical setting, many people can learn biofeedback techniques and continue practicing them at home. Devices that monitor heart rate variability, skin conductance, or muscle tension are becoming more accessible, allowing individuals to practice relaxation techniques and monitor their progress.

Some at-home biofeedback techniques include:

Progressive muscle relaxation: This involves tensing and then relaxing different muscle groups, helping to release physical tension and reduce pain.

Deep breathing exercises: Biofeedback can help individuals recognize when their breathing is shallow or rapid due to stress, and teach them to shift to slow, deep breaths, which calm the nervous system and reduce pain.

Guided visualization: By using biofeedback to observe how the body responds to mental imagery, individuals can learn how positive or calming thoughts influence physical relaxation and pain levels.

Biofeedback requires consistent practice, but over time, individuals can develop greater awareness and control over their body's responses, leading to reduced pain and improved emotional well-being.

CHAPTER SEVEN

LONG-TERM MANAGEMENT OF CHRONIC PAIN

Building a Pain Management Plan

A personalized pain management plan is essential for anyone living with chronic pain. This plan should take into account the underlying cause of your pain, your physical and emotional health, and your lifestyle. The goal is to create a strategy that integrates multiple therapies—both medical and non-medical—so you can manage pain in a way that is both effective and sustainable.

How to Create a Personalized Strategy for Living with Pain

The first step in building a pain management plan is understanding your specific needs and goals. Your plan should address not only your physical pain but also how pain affects your mood, energy levels, sleep, and ability to function in daily life. Key components of a successful pain management plan include:

Medical treatments: This includes medications, injections, or any other medical interventions prescribed by your doctor. These should be tailored to your specific pain condition and adjusted as needed.

Physical activity: Regular, low-impact exercise, such as walking, swimming, or yoga, is crucial for maintaining mobility and reducing stiffness. A physical therapist can help you develop a safe exercise regimen that fits your abilities and limitations.

Psychological support: Pain often takes an emotional toll, and addressing your mental health is just as important as managing physical symptoms. Cognitive Behavioral Therapy (CBT), mindfulness, and other mental health support systems can help you cope with the emotional aspects of living with pain.

Alternative therapies: Complementary approaches like acupuncture, massage therapy, and biofeedback can enhance your pain management efforts by addressing both physical and mental aspects of pain.

Self-care: Learning relaxation techniques, prioritizing sleep, and managing stress are essential to keeping your pain in check and improving your overall well-being.

By combining these elements, you can create a comprehensive plan that addresses all facets of chronic pain and allows for flexibility as your condition changes.

The Role of Your Pain Management Team: Doctors, Therapists, and Specialists

Effective pain management often requires a multidisciplinary team of healthcare providers who can offer different perspectives and treatments. Each member of your pain management team plays a vital role in helping you manage your pain and live a fulfilling life.

Primary care physician: Your primary doctor serves as the coordinator of your pain management plan, ensuring that all treatments are aligned with your overall health and well-being. They can prescribe medications, monitor your progress, and refer you to specialists when necessary.

Pain specialists: These doctors specialize in diagnosing and treating chronic pain conditions. They may offer advanced therapies like nerve blocks, spinal cord stimulators, or other interventions that can reduce pain when traditional treatments aren't enough.

Physical therapists: Physical therapists help you regain strength, flexibility, and mobility. They can teach you exercises that improve your physical functioning without exacerbating your pain.

Mental health professionals: Psychologists or counselors can help you navigate the emotional challenges of chronic pain. Cognitive Behavioral Therapy (CBT), Acceptance and Commitment Therapy (ACT), and other mental health interventions can significantly improve your coping mechanisms.

Alternative therapy practitioners: Acupuncturists, massage therapists, chiropractors, and biofeedback specialists offer complementary treatments that can enhance pain relief and improve your overall quality of life.

Tracking Your Progress

Monitoring your pain and how it responds to various treatments is essential for long-term pain management. Keeping detailed records can help you and your healthcare team identify patterns, adjust treatments, and make informed decisions about what's working and what needs to be changed.

Keeping a Pain Journal to Monitor What Works for You

A pain journal is a valuable tool for tracking your daily pain levels, symptoms, and how different treatments affect your condition. By documenting your experiences, you can gain insights into what triggers flare-ups and which strategies provide relief.

In your pain journal, you should note:

Pain intensity: Rate your pain on a scale of 1 to 10, with 1 being mild discomfort and 10 being unbearable pain. This helps you track fluctuations in your pain levels.

Location of pain: Record where you feel pain, as this can help identify if your pain is spreading or localizing in specific areas.

What activities you did that day: Note any activities, exercises, or movements that may have affected your pain.

Medications and treatments used: List any medications or therapies you used that day, including dosages and how effective they were at reducing pain.

Sleep quality: Record how well you slept, as poor sleep can worsen pain and fatigue.

Mood and energy levels: Chronic pain can affect your mood and mental health, so tracking your emotional state is important.

Tools for Tracking Pain, Symptoms, and Medication

In addition to a pain journal, there are various apps and digital tools designed to help individuals with chronic pain track their symptoms. These tools allow you to monitor pain intensity, track medications, and set reminders for treatments. They can also generate reports that you can share with your healthcare provider, helping to fine-tune your pain management plan.

Some useful tools include:

Pain tracking apps: Apps like Manage My Pain, CatchMyPain, and PainScale allow you to track pain, medications, and triggers in a convenient, digital format.

Wearable devices: Wearables like fitness trackers or smartwatches can help monitor physical activity, sleep patterns, and heart rate, all of which are important for managing chronic pain.

Medication trackers: Keeping track of your medication schedule is crucial, especially if you're taking multiple medications. Apps like Medisafe can help you stay organized and ensure you're following your doctor's instructions.

Adjusting Your Plan Over Time

Chronic pain often changes over time, either because of fluctuations in your condition or the effects of treatments. It's essential to review your pain management plan regularly and make adjustments as needed. Pain management isn't static, and being flexible with your approach can help you stay ahead of changes in your symptoms.

How to Adapt Your Treatments as Your Pain Changes

As your pain evolves, you may need to adjust your treatments. For instance, you might find that certain medications become less effective, or that your body responds better to alternative therapies over time. Regular check-ins with your healthcare team allow for timely adjustments to your pain management plan.

You may need to adapt your treatments if you experience:

Increased pain: If your pain intensifies or becomes more widespread, your doctor may need to adjust your medication dosages, try a different medication, or recommend more advanced therapies like injections or nerve blocks.

Side effects: If you experience side effects from medications, such as fatigue, nausea, or cognitive issues, your doctor may switch you to a different drug or lower the dosage.

Changes in physical ability: If you notice changes in your ability to move or exercise, a physical therapist may adjust your exercise routine to accommodate your needs.

Emotional changes: Increased anxiety, depression, or frustration can affect your pain levels. If you're struggling emotionally, your healthcare team may recommend additional psychological support or therapies like CBT.

Working with Your Doctor to Modify Your Approach as Needed

Effective pain management requires a collaborative approach with your healthcare providers. Regular communication with your doctor allows you to address any new symptoms, concerns, or side effects that arise. Don't hesitate to advocate for yourself and ask for changes if your current treatments aren't working as expected.

Your doctor may suggest:

Rotating medications: To avoid developing tolerance or dependence, some patients benefit from rotating different types of pain medications.

Increasing or decreasing dosages: If your pain worsens or improves, adjusting the dosage of your medications may help maintain effective pain control.

Adding new therapies: As new treatments and therapies become available, your doctor may introduce options that offer better relief or fewer side effects than your current regimen.

CHAPTER EIGHT

COPING WITH THE EMOTIONAL IMPACT OF PAIN

Chronic pain doesn't just affect the body—it also takes a profound toll on emotional and mental health. Living with pain day in and day out can lead to feelings of frustration, helplessness, sadness, and anxiety. It's common for people with chronic pain to experience emotional ups and downs as they navigate the challenges of living with an invisible, ongoing condition. Learning to cope with these emotional struggles is as important as managing the physical pain itself, and doing so can help improve overall quality of life.

Dealing with Emotional Ups and Downs

One of the most difficult aspects of chronic pain is the unpredictability of pain flare-ups and how they can impact mood and emotional stability. Even when pain is well managed, it's natural to experience emotional highs and lows as you adjust to living with an ongoing condition. These emotional shifts are a normal response to chronic pain, but they can be challenging to cope with, especially on days when pain feels overwhelming.

How to Cope When Pain Feels Overwhelming

When pain becomes intense, it can be easy to feel emotionally defeated or discouraged. In these moments, it's important to have strategies in place to help manage both the physical and emotional intensity of the experience. Here are some approaches to consider:

Practice self-compassion: Be gentle with yourself during difficult moments. It's normal to feel frustrated, angry, or sad when pain flares up, but try to remind yourself that you're doing the best you can in a challenging situation.

Focus on what you can control: When pain is severe, it can feel like everything is out of your hands. Ground yourself by focusing on the things you can control—whether it's taking medication, practicing relaxation techniques, or finding a comfortable position to rest in.

Use mindfulness: Mindfulness techniques can help you stay present in the moment and prevent your mind from spiraling into negative thoughts. By focusing on your breath, body sensations, or calming visualizations, you can create some mental space between yourself and the pain.

Break tasks into smaller steps: When pain feels overwhelming, even everyday tasks can seem impossible. Breaking activities into smaller, more manageable steps can help you maintain a sense of control without becoming emotionally overwhelmed.

Reach out for support: Don't hesitate to call a friend, family member, or therapist when you're feeling emotionally drained by pain. Simply talking through your feelings with someone who understands can provide comfort and relief.

Building a Positive Mindset in the Face of Chronic Pain

While it's natural to experience negative emotions due to chronic pain, cultivating a positive mindset can help improve your overall emotional resilience. This doesn't mean ignoring the pain or pretending it doesn't exist, but rather learning to focus on the aspects of life that bring you joy and meaning, even in the face of challenges.

Practice gratitude: Focusing on the things you're grateful for can shift your mindset away from the pain and toward the positives in your life. This could be as simple as acknowledging the support of loved ones or appreciating small pleasures like a warm cup of tea.

Celebrate small victories: Living with chronic pain can make it easy to feel like progress is slow or nonexistent. Acknowledge and celebrate even the smallest victories— whether it's completing a task despite the pain, improving your coping skills, or having a good day after a stretch of bad ones.

Focus on your strengths: Chronic pain can make it easy to feel defeated, but it's important to remember your strengths. Take stock of your personal resilience, perseverance, and ability to adapt to difficult situations.

Finding Emotional Support

Living with chronic pain can feel isolating, particularly if friends or family members don't fully understand the challenges you face. However, finding emotional support—whether through support groups, online communities, or therapy—can make a world of difference in coping with the mental toll of pain.

The Role of Support Groups and Talking with Others Who Understand

One of the most effective ways to find emotional support is by connecting with others who share similar experiences. Support groups, whether in-person or online, offer a safe space to talk openly about your struggles with pain, share coping strategies, and feel understood by people who truly get what you're going through.

Support groups can provide:

Validation: Simply knowing that others are going through the same thing can reduce feelings of isolation and make you feel less alone.

Practical advice: Members of support groups often share tips and strategies that have worked for them, giving you new tools to try in managing your pain.

Emotional relief: Being able to talk about your pain with others who understand can help release pent-up frustration, sadness, or anger.

Connecting with Chronic Pain Communities

Finding Support Groups, Online Forums, and Resources

There are numerous ways to connect with others who are living with chronic pain. Support groups are often hosted by hospitals, pain clinics, or community health organizations. These in-person groups provide a regular space for people to meet, share their experiences, and learn new coping strategies.

For those who prefer the flexibility of virtual connections, online forums and social media groups offer a convenient way to stay connected. Online communities can be particularly beneficial for individuals who have mobility limitations or who live in rural areas where in-person support groups may be limited.
Some popular online chronic pain communities include:

Reddit forums: Subreddits like "r/chronicpain" or "r/fibromyalgia" offer spaces where individuals can ask questions, share experiences, and provide support to one another.

Facebook groups: Many chronic pain communities exist on Facebook, where members can post updates, share articles, and offer advice.

Specialized websites: Websites like PainSupport and MyChronicPainTeam offer resources, forums, and communities specifically for individuals living with chronic pain.

These online platforms provide access to a wealth of knowledge and support that can help you feel more connected and informed about managing your condition.

How to Use Technology to Stay Connected with People Who Understand

Technology has made it easier than ever to stay connected with people who understand your journey. Whether you're using social media, messaging apps, or online forums, you can access a world of support from the comfort of your home. Here's how to use technology to stay connected:

Join online communities: As mentioned earlier, online forums and support groups can be an invaluable source of connection. Use these platforms to ask questions, share your experiences, or simply vent on days when pain feels overwhelming.

Use video calls to stay in touch: Video calls through platforms like Zoom or Skype can help you stay in touch with friends, family, or support group members even if you're unable to leave home. Seeing familiar faces can be a great way to combat feelings of isolation.

Attend virtual support group meetings: Many chronic pain support groups now offer virtual meetings, allowing you to participate from anywhere. These meetings often provide educational resources, group discussions, and the opportunity to share your experiences in a supportive environment.

Stay updated with apps and podcasts: There are also apps and podcasts designed to help individuals with chronic pain stay informed and connected. Apps like MyPainDiary or

PainScale allow you to track your symptoms while offering access to pain management resources.

How to Share Your Experience with Friends and Family

While it's helpful to connect with people who understand chronic pain firsthand, it's also important to maintain open communication with friends and family. Sharing your experience with loved ones helps them better understand what you're going through and offers them the opportunity to provide support.

When talking to friends or family about your pain:
Be honest: It's okay to let loved ones know when you're struggling, even if you don't want to burden them. People who care about you want to support you, but they can't do that if they don't understand what you're going through.

Set boundaries: If you need time to rest or can't participate in certain activities due to pain, communicate your needs clearly. Setting boundaries helps loved ones understand your limitations without feeling rejected.

Educate them: Chronic pain can be difficult for others to grasp, especially if it's invisible. Educating friends and family about your condition can help them better empathize and offer more informed support.

Working with a Therapist

In many cases, working with a therapist can be an essential component of managing the emotional impact of chronic pain. Therapy provides a safe space to explore your feelings, develop coping strategies, and work through the emotional challenges that come with living with pain.

Why Mental Health Counseling Can Be Important for People with Chronic Pain

Chronic pain often leads to a range of emotional struggles, including depression, anxiety, anger, and frustration. Mental health counseling can help address these emotional challenges, providing tools to improve both emotional resilience and pain management.

Therapy can help by:

Addressing negative thought patterns: Cognitive Behavioral Therapy (CBT), for example, helps individuals reframe negative thoughts about pain and build healthier emotional responses.

Developing coping strategies: A therapist can guide you through relaxation techniques, mindfulness practices, and other strategies that reduce stress and improve emotional regulation.

Improving communication: Therapy can also help you learn how to communicate more effectively with loved ones, doctors, or employers about your pain, setting clear boundaries and expressing your needs.

In addition to providing emotional support, therapy can help you navigate the challenges of living with a chronic condition, empowering you to feel more in control of your mental and emotional health.

Finding a Therapist Who Specializes in Chronic Pain

Not all therapists are trained to work with individuals dealing with chronic pain, so finding a therapist who specializes in this area is important. Look for professionals with experience in pain psychology, health psychology, or rehabilitation psychology. These specialists understand the unique mental and emotional challenges faced by people with chronic pain and can tailor therapy to your specific needs.

CONCLUSION

Living Well with Chronic Pain

How to Focus on Quality of Life Despite Pain

Focusing on quality of life requires balancing the need for rest and recovery with the desire to engage in fulfilling activities. Here are some strategies to help you focus on quality of life despite pain:

Prioritize activities that bring joy: Whether it's spending time with loved ones, pursuing hobbies, or exploring nature, make time for things that make you happy and help you feel connected to life beyond your pain.

Set realistic goals: Break larger tasks into smaller, manageable steps, and celebrate each achievement. Setting goals that are within your reach can help you feel productive and fulfilled, even when your pain levels fluctuate.

Manage your energy: Chronic pain can be exhausting, so learn to pace yourself and conserve energy for activities that are most important to you. Don't be afraid to rest when you need it.

Practice self-compassion: Be kind to yourself when things are tough. Chronic pain can be emotionally draining, but treating yourself with patience and understanding can reduce feelings of frustration or guilt.

Tips for Staying Positive and Finding Joy in Everyday Moments

Mindfulness: Incorporate mindfulness practices into your daily routine. Even a few minutes of focused breathing or meditation can help shift your attention away from pain and toward the present moment.

Celebrate small wins: Whether it's getting out of bed, finishing a task, or managing to exercise, acknowledge your achievements—no matter how small.

Surround yourself with positivity: Engage with people, activities, and environments that uplift and inspire you. This can reduce stress and help shift your mindset toward positivity.

Focus on what you can control: Chronic pain can often feel overwhelming because so much of it is outside your control. Focus on the aspects of life you can influence—your mindset, your daily activities, and how you react to challenges.

Moving Forward

Building a Future Where Pain Doesn't Control You

You have the ability to shape your future, even when chronic pain is part of the picture. By managing your condition proactively, seeking out new treatments, and focusing on personal growth, you can create a future where pain is not the central focus. Commit to living a life filled with meaning, connection, and joy, despite the challenges of pain.

Celebrating Your Progress and Resilience

Living with chronic pain takes tremendous strength and resilience. Take the time to reflect on your journey and celebrate the progress you've made. Every step you've taken toward better managing your pain is worth acknowledging. You are stronger than your pain, and your resilience is a testament to your ability to overcome challenges.

Appendices

Glossary of Pain Management Terms

Acupuncture: A traditional Chinese medicine technique that involves inserting thin needles into specific points on the body to relieve pain and promote healing.

Biofeedback: A method that uses sensors to help you gain awareness of and control over physiological functions, such as muscle tension or heart rate, to reduce pain and stress.

Cognitive Behavioral Therapy (CBT): A form of therapy that helps individuals change negative thought patterns and behaviors that can exacerbate pain.

Chronic Pain: Pain that lasts for more than three to six months, persisting beyond the usual course of recovery.

Neuromodulation: A technique that uses electrical impulses to modify nerve activity, often used to relieve chronic pain.

Opioids: A class of strong prescription pain medications that can be effective but carry the risk of addiction and other side effects.

Transcutaneous Electrical Nerve Stimulation (TENS): A therapy that uses low-voltage electrical currents to relieve pain by disrupting pain signals.

Mindfulness: A mental practice that involves paying attention to the present moment without judgment, often used to reduce stress and pain.

Physical Therapy: A therapeutic approach that involves exercises and hands-on treatments to improve mobility, strength, and function while managing pain.

Platelet-Rich Plasma (PRP): A treatment that uses a concentration of platelets from your own blood to promote healing and reduce pain in injured tissues.

Resources for Chronic Pain

Websites, Books, and Organizations to Help You Find Support

Websites:

• **American Chronic Pain Association (ACPA):** Offers resources, support groups, and educational materials for individuals living with chronic pain (www.theacpa.org).

• **PainScale:** Provides pain tracking tools, resources, and a community of support (www.painscale.com).

• **National Institute of Neurological Disorders and Stroke (NINDS):** Offers information on pain research, treatments, and clinical trials (www.ninds.nih.gov).

Books:

• **The Pain Survival Guide:** How to Reclaim Your Life by Dennis C. Turk and Frits Winter: A practical guide for managing chronic pain through a combination of therapies.

• **Explain Pain by David Butler and G. Lorimer Moseley:** A book that breaks down the science of pain and offers strategies for managing it.

Organizations:

• **American Pain Society:** An organization dedicated to research and education in the field of pain management.

- **The National Pain Foundation:** Provides resources and support for individuals dealing with chronic pain.

Tracking Tools

Even Pain Journals, Apps, and Other Tools to Help You Stay on Top of Your Pain Management

Pain Journals: A pain journal allows you to track your pain levels, medications, and any triggers or activities that affect your symptoms. You can write down how your pain fluctuates throughout the day and what helps or worsens it.

Apps:

• **MyPainDiary:** An app that helps you track your pain, medications, and activities, providing reports that you can share with your doctor.

• **PainScale:** This app offers tools for tracking pain, accessing treatment resources, and connecting with a community of chronic pain sufferers.

• **Flaredown:** A symptom-tracking app designed for people with chronic conditions, helping you track symptoms, triggers, and treatments over time.

Other Tools:

• **Wearable devices:** Fitness trackers and other wearable devices can help you monitor your physical activity, sleep patterns, and heart rate, providing insights into how these factors affect your pain.

www.ingramcontent.com/pod-product-compliance
Lightning Source LLC
Chambersburg PA
CBHW071223260726
48653CB00042B/1812